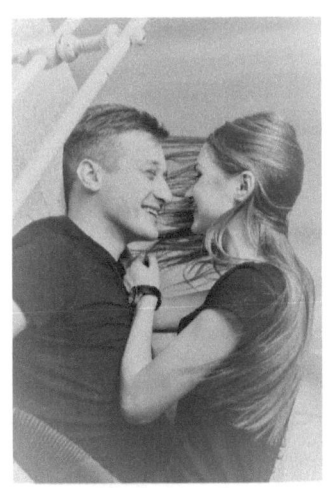

Turn Pages to Get Rid of Obesity AND   Live your Life with Toned Body, Flat Stomach, Glowing Skin & Silky Hair …………… All with No Compromise of feasting your body with your favorite Dishes!!!

the
LEAN
code

OFELDA GARCIA

ZenK Publishing

Copyright Information

Notice

The information presented in this book is not intended for treatment or prevention of obesity or any other disorder. But it tries to explain a proven method to get rid of obesity and other such other disorders However readers are requested to consult your physician before starting any diet or training program.

THE SOUL CALL

"The Secret of Success in Life is to Eat what you like and let the Food fight it out inside"

If only Mark Twain was from our time, he would understand the complexity of his above quote.

Right?

I mean letting the food fight from inside?

Ok maybe it was possible in the '80s and the '90s but in today's life, it is a very controversial quote.

There is a belief that if you want shaped physique, follow the inverted pyramid meal pattern.

Eat breakfast like a king, lunch like a prince and dinner like a pauper.

So, follow this and you will achieve a perfectly shaped body throughout your life.

Case closed?

Hold on...

Maybe that's just one person who did this research and came to this conclusion because his body is built to follow that pattern. What if there are other studies that show skipping meals can be ideal too? I never had my breakfast between 8 to 9 and mostly have brunch and I'm not complaining!

When it comes to the individual body, there is no way a single diet routine be helpful be it   a Keto diet or Vegan diet or Weight Watchers diet. The fast-paced life that we live gives us a very small window to take out time for ourselves. And diet for that matter needs a lot of dedication and sacrifice.

People who are struggling with weight loss are aware of the seriousness of the issue. **Obesity** is a serious medical condition that can cause complications such as metabolic syndrome, high blood pressure, atherosclerosis, heart disease, diabetes, high blood cholesterol, cancers, and sleep disorders. In our day to day life, being obese have a tremendous effect which can be very relatable. Skin-related problems, the stretch marks, itchy skin and so on. Finding that perfect fit for any kind of clothing can be very frustrating, as is having to settle with whatever that fits. The struggle is real and as much as one enjoys being a little lazy or loves the cheese filled pizza crust, it comes with a cost. A rather heavy one.

Irrespective of gender, everyone wishes to have a body to flaunt. A toned upper body, perfect facial cut, shaped thighs (uh hello tanned too.) and most importantly to fit into those jaw-dropping, skin-kissing dresses that are so fabulously hung over a mannequin that doesn't even do justice to the dress. Now don't start to think I'm all into outer beauty. I also do believe what's good inside is better than what's outside. So, shall we talk about that too? I mean one can go on and on over the benefit of being healthy and what dramatic and drastic effects it can have on one's life. Feeling good about yourself every morning just by looking in the mirror can be a huge achievement. Cutting down that medical bill expense which otherwise will go into getting supplements is another satisfaction. When you enjoy that walk in the park for several hours just to relax and not for counting steps on your smartwatch, that is where everyone wants to be. What I'm trying to picture here is being fit is not only a physical deal but comes with a lot of mental peace.

The modern dietary pattern of an average American is generally characterized by high intakes of red meat, processed meat, pre-packaged foods, butter, fried foods, high-fat dairy products, eggs, refined grains, potatoes, corn (and high fructose corn syrup) and high-sugar which literally mean CARBS and SUGAR.

This heavy oil and fat consumption are causing our bodies to take a shape that is not sustainable to survive. There are more **obese** US adults than those who are just **overweight**. According to a study in The Journal of the **American** Medical Association (JAMA), in 2008, the **obesity rate** among adult **Americans** was estimated at 32.2% for men and 35.5% for women; these **rates** were roughly confirmed by the CDC again for 2009–2010.

You see the reason I quoted Mark Twain at the beginning is that he made it very simple to understand a very complex system on how to be healthy. I present the new age version of his quote:

"Let the food fight for you from the inside."

It's just like taking a vacation. When you work too much and exhaust yourself, you need some time away from all the hustle bustle, rejuvenate yourself and come back to normal. It's all about that - our bodies have built in natural course correction systems, we only need to make use of them! The high carb intake in our body is just like us working day and night till the point of exhaustion. Like us, our body too needs to rest a bit and then force start again. In this article, I'm not going to tell you 10 steps to be healthy, I'm not even sure how many steps are there and who cares? Neither I'm going to tell you whether you should lose fat or something. It's a personal choice. But giving the body what it needs is something that we should religiously follow.

If you have been struggling with weight loss all your life, **Intermittent Fasting** can HELP, but it needs to be part of a well-balanced approach that works for your lifestyle, body type, experience, and goals.

A big problem with **Intermittent Fasting** is knowing how to make it work for YOUR life. Depending on when you work, when you exercise if you have a family to prepare meals for, it can get tricky to navigate. Not to mention that Intermittent Fasting is just a piece of the puzzle – you also need to eat better and make exercise a priority!

Now, those are not problems. The real problem is how much you know about **Intermittent Fasting!** And it's just a matter of time when you know what it is and how to implement in your life. And this book exists so you get to know all you need about it, and let it help you live better!

Intermittent fasting is not a diet, but rather a *dieting pattern*.

In simpler terms: it's making a conscious decision to skip certain meals on purpose.

By fasting and then feasting on purpose, intermittent fasting generally means that you consume your calories during a specific window of the day and choose not to eat food for a larger window of time.

There are a few different ways to take advantage of intermittent fasting that we will explore in the latter part of the book.

LET'S GET STARTED!

GO GO OBESE

One Last time let us see what Obese is and go through the life challenges face by them...

Pardon me for terming obesity as a scum because it is a crippling problem for the American populace as we all know from recent statics data that over 160million Americans are either Obese or Overweight. That is 37.9% for men and 41.1% for women according to CDC (Centre for Disease Control and Prevention) as of 2015/2016. According to OECD (Organization for Economic Co-operation and Development), The United States has increased from 23% obesity in 1962 to 57.6% in 2013; What a staggering increment of 33.4%! With this current rate it is estimated that 3 out of 4 people in the United States will be Obese in 2020, this is frightening and very scary and as of such we need to provide a lasting solution to solving this problem with Intermittent fasting as the best of all alternatives.

Before I get into the solution which is "Intermittent fasting", let's enlighten ourselves a bit more on what Obesity really is and the challenges faced by Obese people in the United States. Allow me to take you on a journey of enlightenment, shall we!

WHAT IS OBESITY?

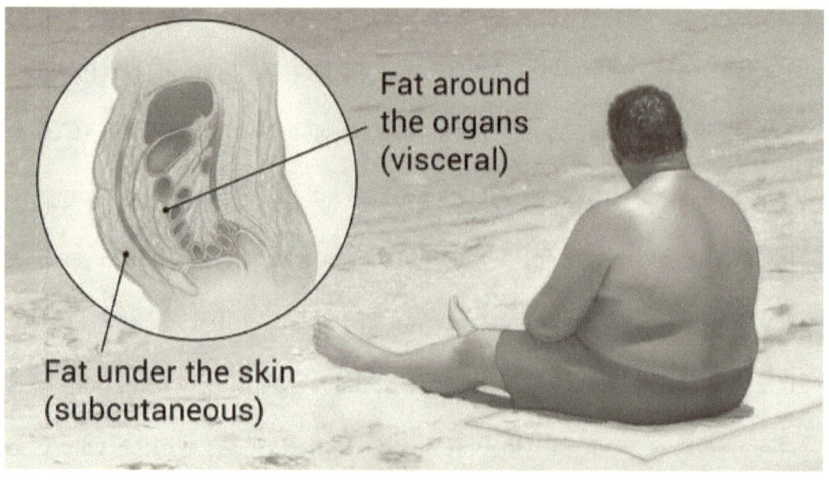

I can imagine that even for a novice the word "Obesity" may not be a mystery (The word itself sounds robust) but what really is this Obesity and at what point of weight gain can we say a person is Obese.

Well, according to a definition provided by MedicalNewsToday, *Obesity is a medical condition that occurs when a person carries excess weight or body fat that might affect their health*. A person with obesity is said to have a High Body Mass Index (BMI). BMI is what doctors use to describe the normal expected body weight for a person of a certain age, sex and weight. A BMI of 25 to 29.9 indicates that a person is carrying excessive weight while a BMI of more than 30 shows that a person is Obese. BMI is a person's weight (in kilograms) divided by the square of his or her height (in meters).

Let's put it this way, my body mass is the expected weight of any person of my age, sex and height. So, if you're a man and you're 35 years old, your BMI is supposed to be around 18.5kg to 24.5kg per meter square, if your BMI is less it means you are underweight, and more BMI means you are overweight.

BMI	Weight status
Below 18.5	Underweight

BMI	Weight status
18.5-24.9	Normal
25.0-29.9	Overweight
30.0-34.9	Obese (Class I)
35.0-39.9	Obese (Class II)
40.0 and higher	Extreme obesity (Class III)

Waist to hip ratio (WHR, this basically means how fat a person's waist is compared to their hip), waist to height ratio (WTHR, this is the fatness of a person's waist compared to their height) and fat distribution in the body can also be used to determine if a person is obese or not.

It's simple, if you see a 10-year-old boy/girl that looks very much fatter than other kids in their peer group it simply means the boy/girl is obese, although obesity should not be mistaken for being muscular or robust.

If you can imagine that obesity comes along with a lot of adverse effects to the immune system, your imagination is just right! Obesity and excess weight can increase the risk of developing several health conditions, including metabolic syndrome, arthritis, and some types of cancer. Metabolic syndrome that can arise from obesity and excess weight includes a collection of issues, such as high blood pressure, type 2 diabetes and cardiovascular diseases.

Here are 10 facts about obesity in the United States.

1.　More than one-third (1 in 3) of adults in the United States are obese.

In the United States, 36.5% of adults are obese. And generally, 32.5% of adults in the United States are overweight. Would you believe that more than two-thirds of adults in the United States are overweight or obese, that's 2 out of 3 people

There many causes of obesity and excess weight, we will discuss majority of these causes subsequently.

2.   Obese children are more likely to grown into obese adults.

Children who are overweight or obese have been found to be five times more likely to become obese or overweight adults than children of normal weight. This can increase their risk for many chronic diseases and health complications.

3.   Obesity is linked to more than 60 chronic diseases.

If you are overweight or obese, your risk for dozens of diseases and conditions is higher. These include type 2 diabetes, heart disease, stroke, cancer, and many other diseases.

4.   Obesity affects 1 in 6 children in the United States.

Around 17% of American children from age 2 to 19 are obese. That's more than 12.7 million American children. One in 8 American preschoolers is obese.

5.   Obesity causes more deaths than being underweight.

Globally, obesity is one of the top 5 leading causes of death. 2.8 million people die yearly due to obesity.

6. The cost of maintaining obesity is high.

Obesity costs Americans $147 billion each year. People who are obese pay more out of pocket than people who are not. In fact, the medical costs for people with obesity are $1,429 higher each year than those of people with a normal weight.

7.   Your waist size increases your risk for diabetes.

Researchers found that men with waist circumferences in the highest 10 % of measurements were 20 times more likely to develop type 2 diabetes than men whose waist circumferences fell in the lowest 10 %. Also, waist measurements may help predict which people with a low or normal weight are more likely to develop diabetes.

8.   Your ethnicity can affect your likelihood of obesity.

Your ethnicity may also affect your risk for obesity. Almost half (48.4 %) of non-Hispanic blacks have obesity. They're followed by Hispanics with 42.6 %, non-Hispanic whites with 36.4%, and non-Hispanic Asians with 12.6 %.

9. All states in America have obesity rates above 20 %.

Would you believe that as of 2017, all 50 states have an obesity rate over 20%? And about 20 years ago, no state in America had a rate above 15%.

10.   Americans are eating more calories than ever before.

Today, Americans eat 23 % more calories than we did in 1970. That can really add up. One of the leading causes of overweight and obesity is an imbalance of calories. When you eat more than you burn, your body stores the extra energy as fat. Over time, the pounds can begin to pile on, we will discuss more about this in the causes of obesity.

CAUSES OF OBESITY

1. Consuming too many calories

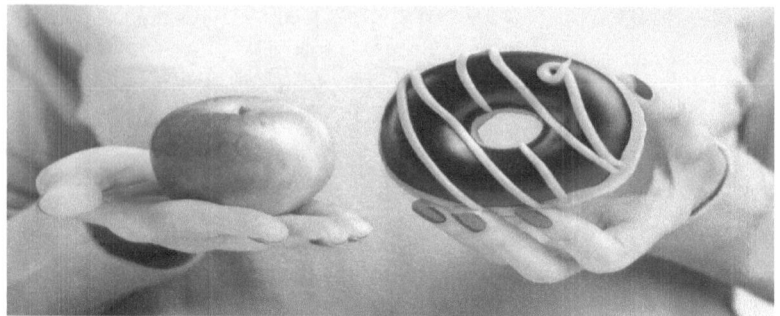

According to "MedicalNewsToday" when a person consumes more calories than they use as energy, their body will store the extra calories as fat. This can lead to excess weight and obesity.

In addition to this, some types of foods are more likely to lead to weight gain, especially those that are high in fats and sugars.

Foods that tend to increase the risk of weight gain include:

- Fast foods

- Fried foods, such as French fries

- Fatty and processed meats

- Dairy products

- Foods with added sugar, such as baked goods, ready-made breakfast cereals, and cookies

- Foods containing hidden sugars, such as ketchup and many other canned and packaged food items

- Sweetened juices, sodas, and alcoholic drinks

- Processed, high-carb foods, such as bread and bagels.

Some processed food products contain high-fructose corn syrup as a sweetener, including savory items, such as ketchup. Eating too much of these foods and doing too little or no exercise can result in weight gain and obesity.

2.   Lack of sleep or not enough sleep

Research has suggested that missing sleep increases the risk of gaining weight and developing obesity. When a person does not sleep enough, their body produces ghrelin, a hormone that stimulates appetite. At the same time, a lack of sleep also results in a lower production of leptin, a hormone that suppresses the appetite. This means that lack of sleep causes you to eat more than normal.

3. Inactivity

If you're not very active, you don't burn as many calories. With a sedentary lifestyle, you can easily take in more calories every day than you use through exercise and normal daily activities.

PS: AVOID HIGH-FRUCTOSE CORN SYRUP

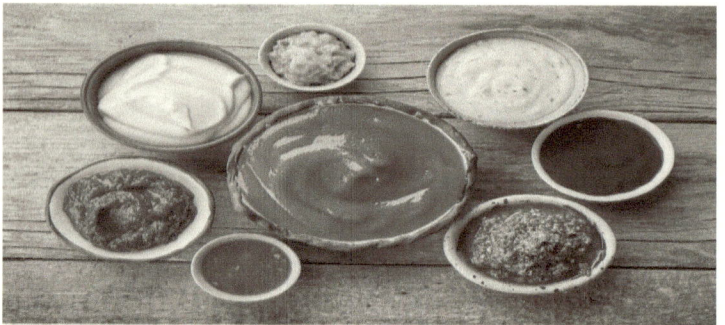

4. Obesity gene

Obesity can also be hereditary, that is it can be passed down from the parents to the child through a faulty gene called the fat-mass and obesity-associated gene (FTO). This is responsible for some cases of obesity.

5.   Medications

Medications associated with weight gain include certain antidepressants (medications used in treating depression), anticonvulsants (medications used in controlling seizures and some diabetes medications), certain hormones such as oral contraceptives.

In a more general sense, let us breakdown some of the adverse effects and disadvantages of Obesity and the challenges faced by Obese people in the United States.

CHALLENGES FACED BY OBESE PEOPLE IN THE UNITED STATES

Excerpts provided by Wikipedia shows that Obesity in the United States is a major health issue, resulting in numerous diseases, specifically significant increase in early mortality and economic costs.

While many industrialized countries have experienced similar increases, **obesity rates in the United States are the highest in the world.**

Obesity causes about 100,000–400,000 deaths in the United States per year.

Obesity has caused an increase in health care use and expenditures, costing the American society an estimated $117 billion in direct and indirect costs. This exceeds health care costs associated with smoking and accounts for 6% to 12% of national health care expenditures in the United States, this indicates that America spends more money on obesity healthcare than that of smokers.

Obesity has also been shown to increase the prevalence of complications during pregnancy and childbirth. Babies born to obese women are almost three times as likely to die within one month of birth and almost twice as likely to be stillborn than babies born to women of normal weight.

Obesity causes a short life-span often reducing the life-span of people with severe obesity by an about 5 to 20 years.

Carrying around extra pounds can create a variety of health problems from causing your joints to ache.

Obesity has also been shown to increase the prevalence of complications during pregnancy and childbirth. Babies born to obese women have been found to be almost three times as likely to die within one month of birth and almost twice as likely to be stillborn than babies born to women of normal weight.

Obesity is also known to cause several potentially serious health problems, including:

- High triglycerides and low high-density lipoprotein (HDL) cholesterol

- Type 2 diabetes

- High blood pressure

- Metabolic syndrome — a combination of high blood sugar, high blood pressure, high triglycerides and low HDL cholesterol

- Heart disease

- Stroke

- Cancer, including cancer of the uterus, cervix, endometrium, ovaries, breast, colon, rectum, esophagus, liver, gallbladder, pancreas, kidney and prostate

- Breathing disorders, including sleep apnea, a potentially serious sleep disorder in which breathing repeatedly stops and starts

- Gallbladder disease

- Gynecological problems, such as infertility and irregular periods

- Erectile dysfunction and sexual health issues

- Nonalcoholic fatty liver disease, a condition in which fat builds up in the liver and can cause inflammation or scarring

- Osteoarthritis

QUALITY OF LIFE

When you're obese, your overall quality of life may be diminished. You may not be able to do things you used to do, such as participating in enjoyable activities. You may avoid public places. Obese people may even encounter discrimination.

Other weight-related issues that may affect your quality of life include:

- Depression

- Disability

- Sexual problems

- A sense of shame and guilt

- Social isolation

- Lower work achievement

Enough is Enough....no more talk of obese...

EMBRACE TONED BODY

Everyone loves how glamour models look slim and stunning in photographs. With flat tummies, great hair and glowing skin. Think about your favorite celebrity, we all want to look as lovely and as stunning as they look. Turn on the television or pick up a glossy magazine and you'll be bombarded with tons of messages that a lean body is beautiful. Well it is!

Let's talk about some of the few reasons why having a normal weight is beneficial to the human health and why it helps to live a positive life.

There are many more reasons to get yourself a healthy weight, if you're not there already. You'll feel more positive, better and have more energy. You'll also drastically lower your chances of having high blood pressure, type 2 diabetes, heart disease, arthritis, and even conditions like sleep apnea. In case you already have health conditions like hypertension or diabetes, weight loss can reduce the severity of the disease.

You don't necessarily have to get the appearance of a model in a magazine to get all the benefits of being at a healthy weight. Losing just a few pounds can make you significantly healthier and more positive about yourself.

Everyone will admit that it's a lovely feeling to wear a skimpy swimsuit and know you look amazing in it. But maintaining a healthy weight (whether that means dropping a few pounds or gaining some) is about so much more than inciting than looking stunning in a swimsuit. Here's a few more reasons a healthy weight rock.

Decreased Breast Cancer Risk: Having a normal weight reduces your proximity and risk to breast cancer by 30 – 60 %.

Improved Heart Health: Having a normal weight prevents the risk to heart attack and other cardiovascular diseases.

Increased Fertility: The American Society for Reproductive Medicine estimates that 12 percent of infertility cases are because of weight-related issues (with roughly an equal number of people suffering from infertility being overweight and underweight). Why is this so? Especially for women your weight can affect your periods and ovulation—so if you're not at a healthy poundage, your fertility can suffer.

Normal weight equals better Sleep: According to a 2012 study from Johns Hopkins University School of Medicine, losing weight especially abdominal fat—can help you log higher-quality sleep. "It becomes harder for the lungs to expand because fat is in the way." And since breathing issues can lead to nighttime problems like sleep apnea, it takes a toll on the amount of sleep you get.

Easier to make clothes fit: With flat abs, you won't have to worry about fitting into your favorite clothes ever again.

A longer lifespan: It's no secret that normal weight people have a lower risk of disease and thus, live longer. It is estimated that the lifespan of an obese person is up to 10 years shorter than that of a normal-weight person. This means a normal weight person lives longer than an obese person.

I can imagine that we all want to live long and have good health, so how do we chow down on some of that weight hindering us. The answer is simple; we need to reduce it. Another question arises, with so many so-called methods available on the internet nowadays, which one is the best method to reduce weight in a healthy manner.

The answer is yet again very simple. INTERMITTENT FASTING.

Before I jump straight into what intermittent fasting is and why it works. Here's a list of popular American celebrities that swore by the practice of Intermittent fasting.

1. **HUGH JACKMAN** popular for playing the role of wolverine in the X-men series. "I haven't put on nearly the amount of fat I normally would. And the great thing about this diet is, I sleep so much better", he said this during an interview

2. **KOURTNEY KARDASHIAN** the eldest of the famous Kardashian sisters. Kourtney Kardashian has been quite vocal about her fasting plan, where she does a 24hour fast one day a week and doesn't eat for 14-16 hours after dinner.

3. **TERRY CREWS** former American football player, fitness model and actor. Terry is said to eat his first meal at 2pm and then have his last at 10pm.

4. **MIRANDA KERR** international model and fitness ambassador

5. **JENNIFER LOPEZ** famous popstar and dancer. She's also known for her curvy physique and shape.

6. **JIMMY KIMMEL** talk show host and producer of Jimmy Kimmel live

7. **CHRIS HEMSWORTH** popular for playing Thor in Marvel's Avengers series.

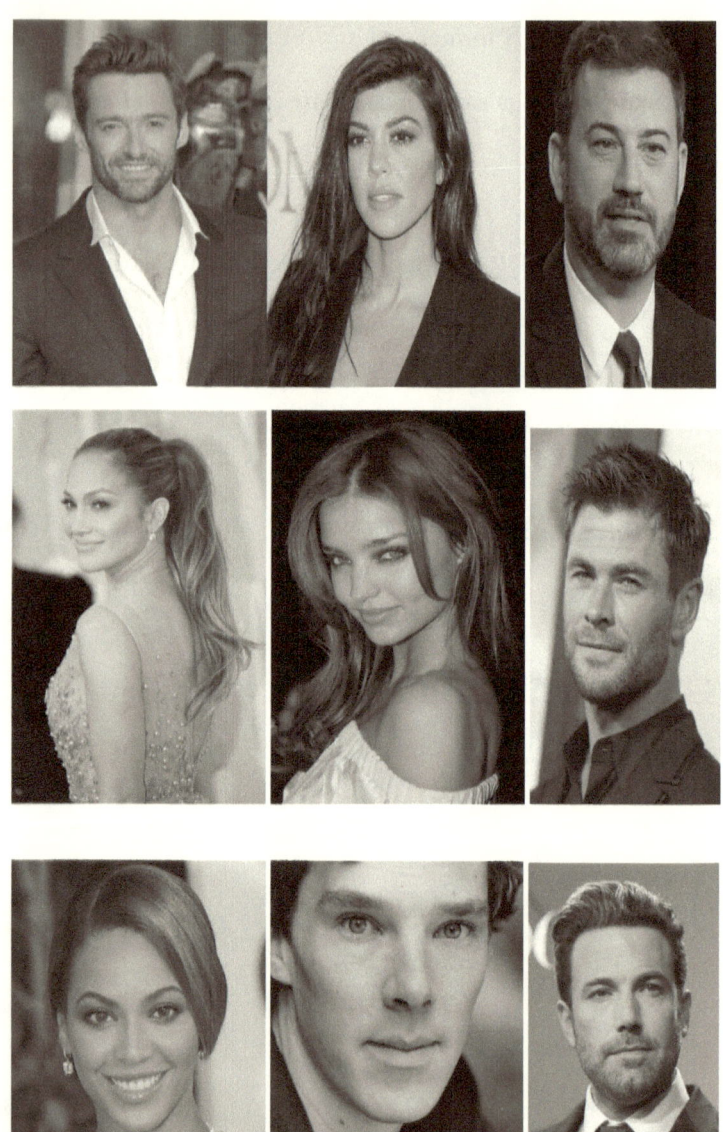

8. BEYONCE KNOWLES-CARTER popular popstar, dancer and multiple Grammy award winner

9. BENEDICT CUMBERBATCH popular for playing Sherlock Holmes and Doctor Strange

10. BEN AFFLECK yep that's Batman

DEFINE INTERMITTENT FASTING

Before We breakdown the concept of Intermittent fasting let's starts by understanding the two words that form the concept.

The word "Intermittent" according to the Oxford's advanced learners' dictionary, means stopping and starting often over a period but not regularly. Other words that can be used for intermittent include periodic, alternate, shifting, coming and going, recurrent, sporadic, irregular, broken, seasonal, rhythmic, serial, epochal, cyclical, cyclic, discontinuous, interrupted, every other, spasmodic, on and off, fitful, occasional, now and then etc.

The word "fasting" means the act of a fast. A fast can be further defined as the act of eating little to no food due to religious or health reasons.

For the sake of this editorial and write-up, let's assume the definition of fasting as the act of eating no food for a period due to health reasons.

Merging these two words gives us pretty much a straightforward guess of the concept. Intermittent fasting is simply the act of following a start-stop approach to eating.

Let me break it down further for simplicity. Intermittent fasting doesn't mean starvation. Fasting is very different from starvation because starvation is the absence of food for a very long time without control leading to severe pain and sometimes death. Fasting on the other hand can be controlled, it may be stopped at any time a person wants. It's done by someone who is not underweight and thus has enough stored body fat to live off. Intermittent fasting done right should not cause suffering, and certainly never death. Food is easily available, but you choose not to eat it. This can be for any period, from a few hours up to a few days or – with medical supervision – even weeks on end. You may begin a fast at any time of your choosing, and you may end a fast at will, too. You can start or stop a fast for any reason or no reason at all. Fasting has no standard duration, as it is merely the absence of eating.

Anytime that you are not eating, you are intermittently fasting. For example, you may fast between dinner and breakfast the next day, a period of approximately 12-14 hours. In that sense, intermittent fasting should be considered a part of everyday life.

Take for example the word "breakfast". Breakfast refers to the meal that breaks your fast – which is done daily. This is because whenever we sleep we are fasting since we are not eating even if only for a short duration. Intermittent fasting is not difficult to understand so you don't have to be curious, it is a part of everyday, normal life.

Intermittent fasting involves entirely or partially abstaining from eating for a set amount of time, before eating regularly again.

Intermittent fasting is not a diet. It is a timed approach to eating. Unlike a dietary plan that restricts where calories come from, intermittent fasting does not specify what foods a person should eat or avoid.

Although to use intermittent fasting as a solution to obesity, a diet plan may be recommended. Intermittent fasting may have some health benefits, including weight loss but is not suitable for everyone.

Intermittent fasting involves cycling between periods of eating and fasting. At first, people may find it difficult to eat during a short window of time each day or alternate between days of eating and not eating.

Intermittent fasting is currently one of the world's most popular health and fitness trends. It is derived from traditional fasting, a universal ritual used for health or spiritual benefit as described in early texts by Socrates, Plato, and religious groups. Fasting typically entails a steady abstinence of food and beverages, ranging from 12 hours to one month. It may require complete abstinence or allow a reduced amount of food and beverages.

Prolonged very low-calorie diets can cause physiological changes that may cause the body to adapt to the calorie restriction and therefore prevent further weight loss. Intermittent fasting attempts to address this problem by cycling between a low-calorie level for a brief time followed by normal eating.

Intermittent fasting doesn't change *what* you eat, it changes *when* you eat. It's a way of scheduling your meals so that you get the most out of them.

You may be thinking.

How is this possible? Isn't skipping breakfast bad for you? Why would anyone fast for 12-16 hours every day? What are the benefits? Is there any science behind this or are you just crazy? Is it dangerous to starve Yourself?

Take a deep breath. You're not about to do something crazy, and this works. It's easy to implement into your lifestyle and there are tons of health benefits.

How about we dive straight into things? In this write-up, together we will break down intermittent fasting and everything that goes with it.

Let's talk about why intermittent fasting is worth it.

Firstly, wouldn't it be awesome to find a way to lose weight without going on a crazy diet? The truth is many of us love the sweet things in life, many of which are rich in calories and excess sugar cutting. So, wouldn't it be awesome if you could still eat what you want but only when you undergo a period of intermittent fasting? In fact, most of the time you'll try to keep your calories the same when you start intermittent fasting. Additionally, intermittent fasting is a good way to keep muscle mass on while getting lean.

The main reason people try intermittent fasting is to lose fat and reduce obesity. We'll discuss how intermittent fasting leads to fat loss and why it is the best solution to get rid of obesity in a moment.

Intermittent fasting is a simple yet effective strategy for taking bad weight off while keeping good weight on because it requires very little behavior change. This is a very good thing because it means intermittent fasting falls into the category of "simple methods that work. Simple enough that anyone can actually do it, and yet effective enough that it will actually make a difference."

Let's get to a more interesting part. – How Intermittent fasting works to reduce obesity and why it is the best solution to get a toned body!

HOW IF WORKS?

The knowledge of how intermittent fasting works boils down to understanding the difference between the feeding state and the fasting state.

What happens when we feed and what happens when we don't?

In the feeding state the body is digesting and absorbing food. Basically, the feeding state starts when we begin to eat and lasts for 3-5 hours as our body digests and absorbs the food we just ate. Whenever we feed, it's very difficult for our body to burn fat because our insulins are high, and the body keeps producing more for storage in the liver as sugar.

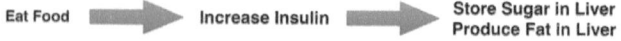

Eat Food → Increase Insulin → Store Sugar in Liver / Produce Fat in Liver

After this process, our body goes into what is known as the post–absorptive state, a state whereby the body stops processing a meal. The post–absorptive state lasts until 8 to 12 hours after your last meal, which is when you enter the fasting state. It is much easier for the body to burn fat in the fasting state because insulin levels are low.

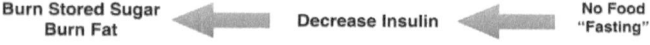

Burn Stored Sugar / Burn Fat ← Decrease Insulin ← No Food "Fasting"

If we start eating the minute we get up from bed, and do not stop until we go to sleep, we spend almost all our time in the feeding state. If we continue this process, there is a huge chance that we may gain weight, because we have not given our body the time to burn the stored food energy. To lose weight or balance the effect of overfeeding, we may simply need to increase the amount of time spent burning food energy. That's intermittent fasting.

The main reason why intermittent fasting works is because it helps you reduce the consumption of calories.

In other words, Intermittent fasting helps to BURN STORED FAT AS ENERGY.

WEIGHT LOSS

Asides from having a cleansing, detoxification and purification effect. The most effective benefit of Intermittent fasting is weight loss. Remember that the goal is to reduce weight to reduce obesity.

Intermittent Fasting helps you to reduce Insulin resistance, lowering your Risk to Type 2 Diabetes which has become incredibly common in recent decades. Its main feature is high blood sugar levels in the context of insulin resistance. Anything that reduces insulin resistance should help lower blood sugar levels and protect against type 2 diabetes. Amazingly, intermittent fasting has been shown to have major benefits for insulin resistance and lead to an impressive reduction in blood sugar levels.

Another benefit of intermittent fasting is that it makes healthy eating simpler. This makes it easier for you to stick to a healthy and nutritious diet in the long run.

In a nutshell the breakdown of the benefits of intermittent fasting include:

• Weight and body fat loss

• Increased fat burning

• Lowered blood insulin and sugar levels

• Possibly reversal of type 2 diabetes

• Possibly improved mental clarity and concentration

• Possibly increased energy

• Possibly increased growth hormone, at least in the short term

• Possibly an improved blood cholesterol profile

• Possibly a reduction in the risk of Alzheimer's disease

• Possibly longer life

• Possibly activation of cellular cleansing by stimulating autophagy

• Possibly reduction of inflammation

Fasting offers many important unique advantages that are not available in typical diets. Where diets can complicate life, intermittent fasting may simplify it. And as discussed earlier, fasting is a potentially powerful method for lowering insulin and decreasing body weight.

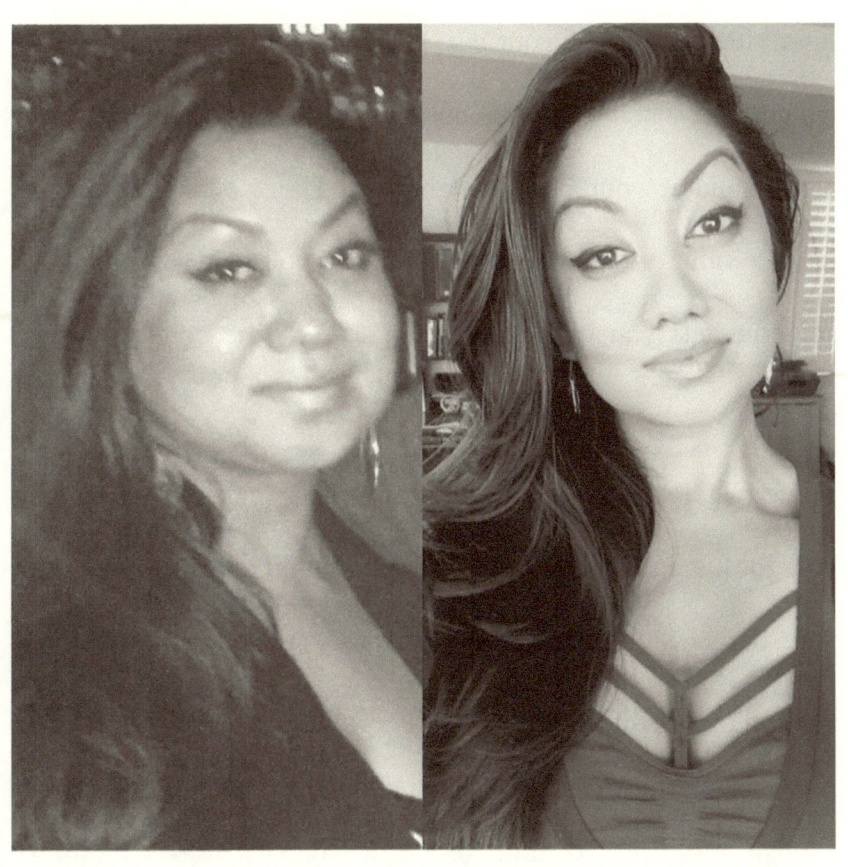

The picture of Sumaya Kazi - Sumaya shared this along with her story of how intermittent fasting changed her life in 2016. In a post she put up in medium.com, she said she lost about 50 pounds of weight in 7 months due to intermittent fasting.

Intermittent fasting is your best bet when considering the perfect weight loss scheme because not only does it reduces body fat, it also regulates your body metabolism. Think of this as getting double value without losing anything, well asides from those stubborn fats you will be shedding. That's the point anyways, isn't it?

To convince you as to why Intermittent fasting works. Imagine you got lost in a desert for one week, the effect of starvation on your body would cause your body to start body excess stored sugar as energy. This excess stored sugar and calorie is FAT. Now let's shun the drastic imagination and forget about starvation for now. Imagine you were placed in a desert with 21 loaves of bread and 14 liters of water as your only option for seven days after which you will be rescued. If we were on the same page, I would say; eat 3 loaves each day and drink 2 liters of water each day, right? Well, many of us if not all will agree to this simple survival scheme even though we might not be all comfortable with it. You will notice a substantial decrease in your body weight after your rescue on the seventh day, this is pretty much how Intermittent fasting works and why it is very much effective.

The desert analogy was a little bit drastic but think about the working process of Intermittent fasting as a procedure of intentionally watching when, how and what you eat to shed weight. It works! And besides you're in full control during the period of intermittent fasting.

I just told you, you are in full control during Intermittent fasting, not some medications, not some plastic surgeon. YOU!

So why not get started by elaborating the different types of Intermittent Fasting and then we will make a step by step plan on how to execute any technique that you would choose.

WHICH IF TYPE SUITS YOU?

1.   Daily Intermittent Fasting: This is also known as the 16/8 schedule or leangains method

This schedule uses a 16–hour fast followed by an 8–hour eating period. This model of daily intermittent fasting was popularized by a fitness expert known as Martin Berkhan of leangains.com. It doesn't matter when you start your 8–hour eating period. You can start at 8am and stop at 4pm. Or you start at 2pm and stop at 10pm. Do whatever works for you. I Myself have found that eating around 1pm and 8pm works well because those times allow me to eat lunch and dinner with friends and family. Breakfast is typically a meal that I eat on my own, so skipping it isn't a big deal.

In this method, you typically eat two or three meals within an 8-hour period.

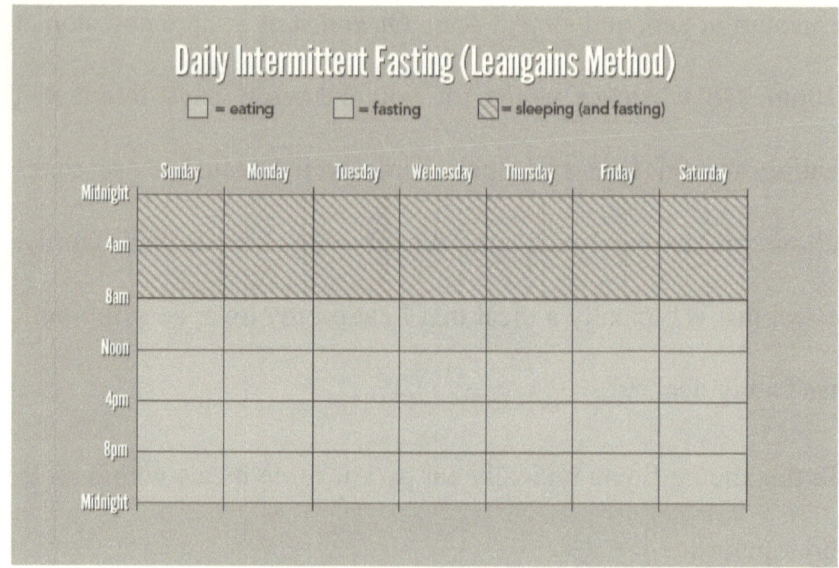

Because daily intermittent fasting is done every day it becomes very easy to get into the habit of eating on this schedule. Right now, you're probably eating around the same time every day without thinking about it. Well, with daily intermittent fasting it's the same thing, you just learn to not eat at certain times, which is remarkably easy because you're in control. One downside of this schedule is that because you typically cut out a meal or two out of your day, and this is OK. Let's simplify this, it's tough to teach yourself to eat bigger meals on a consistent basis. This schedule therefore causes you to lose weight, which is the goal.

2.   Alternate Day Intermittent Fasting: Also known as the 5/2 method

Alternate day intermittent fasting models longer fasting periods on alternating days throughout the week.

Some people fast on alternate days to improve blood sugar, cholesterol, and for weight loss. A person on the 5/2 method typically eats 500 to 600 calories on two non-consecutive days each week. For the rest of the week, such a person will eat only the number of calories they burn during the day. Over time, this creates a calorie deficit that allows the person to lose weight.

For example, in the graphic below you would eat dinner on Monday night and then not eat again until Tuesday evening. On Wednesday, however, you would eat all day and then start the 24–hour fasting cycle again after dinner on Wednesday evening. This allows you to get long fast periods on a consistent basis while also eating at least one meal every day of the week.

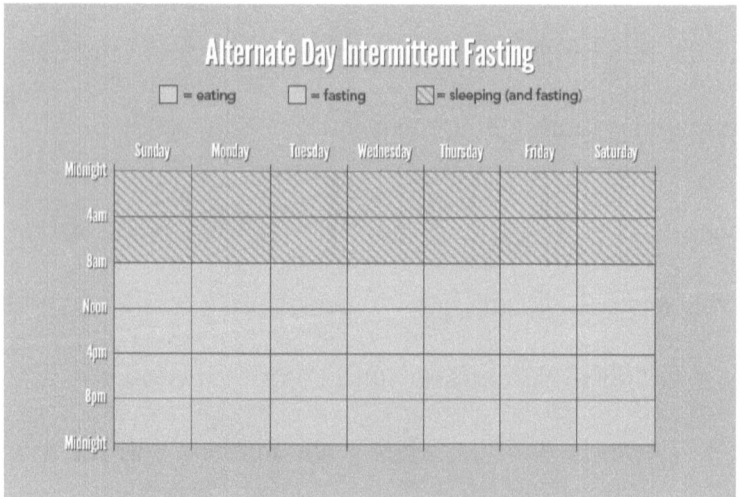

This style of intermittent fasting seems to be popular in research works, but it is not popularly used by people.

The benefit of alternate day intermittent fasting is that it gives you longer time in the fasted state than the Leangains style of fasting. Hypothetically, this would increase the benefits of fasting and drastic weight-loss might occur.

Based on experience, teaching yourself to consistently eat more is one of the harder parts of intermittent fasting. You might be able to feast for a meal but learning to do so every day of the week takes a little bit of planning, a lot of cooking, and consistent eating, so take your time and be steady.

3. Weekly Intermittent Fasting

One of the best ways to get started with intermittent fasting is to do it once per week or once per month. The occasional fast has been shown to lead to many of the benefits of fasting we've already talked about, so even if you don't use it to cut down on calories consistently there are still many other health benefits of fasting.

The illustration below shows one example of how a weekly intermittent fast might play out.

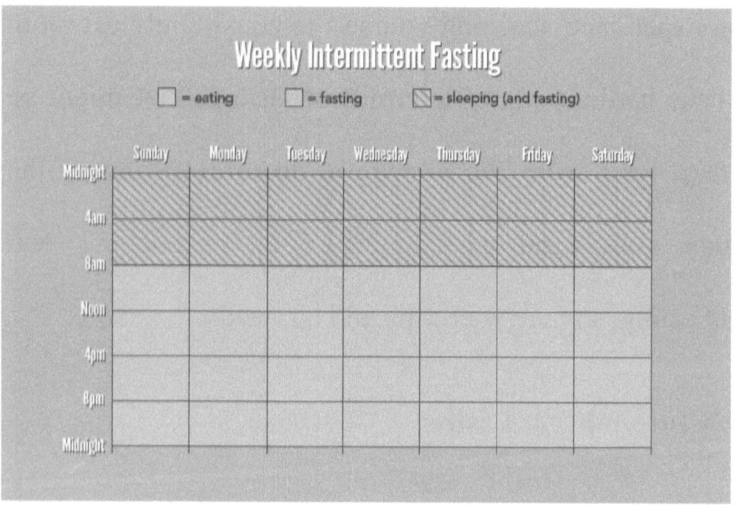

In this example, lunch on Monday is your last meal of the day. You then fast until lunch on Tuesday. This schedule has the advantage of allowing you to eat every day of the week while still reaping the benefits of fasting for 24 hours. This schedule is the least effective for losing weight because you are only cutting out two meals per week. So, if you're looking to lose weight quickly, then this is not your best option.

For a beginner you can also try out the 12/12 method

4.   12:12 Method

Fast for 12 hours a day and eat within a 12-hour window. For example, if you eat your last meal of the day by 8 pm and then wake up to eat breakfast at 8 am you have just completed a 12/12 intermittent fasting cycle. This is simple and often recommended for beginners.

The result is that intermittent fasting results in losing some weight. GUARANTEED!

With this assurance, let's talk about some food/diet plan during

intermittent fasting.

FEAST PLAN

Many dieticians and fitness instructors believe that you can allow yourself to eat anything while doing Intermittent Fasting, including fast food, sugary foods and highly processed dishes. Well, if your goal is to lose weight, if your goal is to improve productivity and if your goal is to simply get healthier, then this believe is wrong. It is important to stick to healthy meals. This means eating whole foods and avoiding foods high in sugar, processed foods, empty carbs etc.

The type of diet you choose is up to you, as long it is balanced and fits your lifestyle. For many people, a healthy diet along with Intermittent Fasting has proven to be very helpful in burning more fat. Let's fix ourselves a good diet plan to fit our chosen intermittent fasting plan. Shall we?

Firstly, let's breakdown a few general foods that you should keep in your fridge/kitchen to succeed in your Intermittent fasting mission.

1.   Water

During your period of fasting, it is important to stay well hydrated. The healthiness and functioning of every major organ in the human body requires proper hydration. Everyone drinks different quantities of water, so I will not be dictating how many liters of water you should drink. Just remember that low water content in the body coupled with limited food could be very injurious to your health. If the thought of plain water doesn't excite you, add a squeeze of lemon juice, a few mint leaves, or cucumber slices to your water. It's still water anyways.

2.   Fish

The Dietary Guidelines suggests eating at least eight ounces of fish per week. Not only are fish rich in healthy fats and protein, it also contains substantial amounts of vitamin D. Since you would be eating only a limited amount of food during your fasting hours, wouldn't it be nice to have a good nutritious ounce of fish to buff up your body system? Not to mention that limiting your calorie intake may take a toll on your brain function, and fish is often considered a very good "brain food."

3.   AVOCADO

Although eating one of the most calorie-rich fruits may not be beneficial to your quest for weight loss, eating a slice or two of avocado is highly nutritious and good for the body. A study even found that adding a half of an avocado to your lunch may keep you full for hours longer than normal.

4.   Nuts

They may be higher in calories than many other snacks, but nuts contain something that most junk food doesn't and that is good fat. I understand that we are trying to get rid of fat but taking a little bit of good fat helps regulate the body metabolism.

5. Eggs

One large egg has six grams of protein and cooks up in minutes. Getting as much protein as possible is important for keeping full and building muscle. One study found that men who ate an egg breakfast instead of a bagel were less hungry and ate less throughout the day. In other words, when you're looking for something to do during your fasting period, why not hard-boil some eggs?

6. Beans and Legumes

I suggest throwing in some low-calorie carbs, like beans and legumes, into your eating plan. Plus, foods like chickpeas, black beans, peas, and lentils have been shown to decrease body weight, even without calorie restriction. Peas are good for you, try them during your fasting period.

7.   Vegetables

Generally, greens such as broccoli, sprouts, and cauliflower are all rich in fiber. When you're going through your fasting period, it's crucial to eat fiber-rich foods that will keep you regular and prevent constipation. Fiber also can make you feel full, which is something you may want if you're fasting for long hours.

8.   Berries

Berries are naturally enriched with vital nutrients. Strawberries for example, are a great source of immune-boosting vitamin C, with more than 100 percent of the daily value in one cup. And that's not even the best part a recent study found that people who consumed a diet rich in flavonoids, like those in blueberries and strawberries, had smaller increases in BMI over a 14-year period than those who did not eat berries. So, I suggest you include some berries in your diet plan for your days of intermittent fasting. To make it even more interesting, try drinking smoothies packed with different types of berries.

9.   Whole Grains

It may seem like being on a diet and eating carbs belong in two different buckets, but not always! Whole grains are rich in fiber and protein and remember that fiber keeps you full. Plus, a new study suggests that eating whole grains instead of refined grains may assist your metabolism. So, feel free to eat your whole grains.

10. Potatoes

Although potatoes contain a slight amount of carb, studies have found potatoes to be one of the most nutritious foods to eat during intermittent fasting. Another study found that eating potatoes as part of a healthy diet could help with weight loss. Although, French fries and potato chips or any fried food in general should be avoided.

I recommend keeping the first two meals of the intermittent fasting meal plan very healthy and small. If you break your fast with a big meal you will be forcing your body to assume that it's not fasting but only went through starvation for a short while. This will not aid in fat burning and it will even make you tired. Moreover, a big meal during the day will cause you to be even more hungry. Lastly cooking, eating and cleaning a large meal during the day is a hassle and is not very lifestyle friendly. With this intermittent fasting diet meal plan, the goal is to eat just enough food to nourish your body and stave off hunger without over-starving your digestive system. This will allow you to reserve your energy and be able to fulfill the fasting period.

To get all the health benefits of Intermittent Fasting such as fat loss, increased metabolic rate, lower blood sugar levels, boost in the immune system and others, you must restrict from consuming any caloric food. But you can still consume non-caloric beverages because they do not break your fast and allow you to get all the benefits of fasting. This is because non-caloric beverages do not cause the release of insulin and therefore, do not interfere with fat burning. During your intermittent fasting period you should drink: Sparkling water, Mineral water, Plain black coffee and Plain tea.

In a more direct way, below is a well-planned diet illustrated for better explanation.

IN SUMMARY: With intermittent fasting, you still need to eat healthy and maintain a calorie deficit if you want to lose weight. Being consistent is crucial, strength training and discipline is important.

With all these being said, intermittent fasting is the most useful tool to lose weight and reduce obesity. It should be recommended for everyone battling with weight gain and obesity. Intermittent fasting is for determined people, people who are ready to exert control over their body and take full responsibility in winning the war against obesity. Remember, self-discipline and control are the keywords for a successful intermittent fasting plan.

STEP BY STEP PLAN THAT SUITS YOU

There are a few different ways to take advantage of intermittent fasting.

16/8 PROTOCOL:

What it is: Fasting for 16 hours and then only eating within a specific 8-hour window. For example, only eating from noon-8 PM, essentially skipping breakfast.

Some people only eat in a 6-hour window or even a 4-hour window. This is "feasting" and "fasting" parts of your days and the most common form of Intermittent Fasting. It's also my preferred method.

24 HOUR PROTOCOL:

Skipping two meals one day, where you are taking 24 hours off from eating. For example, eating on a normal schedule (finishing dinner at 8 PM) and then not eating again until 8 PM the following day.

So, you would eat your normal 3 meals per day, and then occasionally pick a day to skip breakfast and lunch the next day.

If you can only do an 18 hour fast, or a 20 hour fast, or a 22 hour fast – that's okay! Adjust with different time frames and see how your body responds.

Example: Skipping breakfast and lunch one day of the week, and then another where you skip lunch and dinner one day, two days a week.

Note: You can do this once a week, twice a week, or whatever works best for your life and situation.

Those are the two most popular intermittent fasting protocols, though there are many variations of both that you can modify for yourself.

Some people eat in a 4-hour window, others do 6 or 8. Some people do 20-hour fasts or 24-hour fasts. You'll need to experiment with them, adjust them to work for your lifestyle and goals, and see how your body responds.

Let's first get into the science here behind Intermittent Fasting and why you should consider it!

Now, you might be thinking: "okay, so by skipping a meal, I will eat less than I normally eat on average (2 meals instead of 3), and thus I will lose weight, right?"

Yes, by cutting out an entire meal each day, you are consuming fewer calories per week – even if your two meals per day are slightly bigger than before. Overall, you're still consuming fewer calories per day. This is highlighted in a recent JAMA study in which both calorie-restricted dieters and intermittent fasters lost similar amounts of weight over a year period.

Intermittent Fasting can help because your body operates differently when "feasting" compared to when "fasting".

When you eat a meal, your body spends a few hours processing that food, burning what it can from what you just consumed. Because it has all of this readily-available, easy to burn energy (thanks to the food you ate), your body will choose to use that as energy rather than the fat that you have stored. This is especially true if you just consumed carbohydrates/sugar, as your body prefers to burn sugar as energy before any other source.

During the "fasted state" (the hours in which your body is not consuming or digesting any food) your body doesn't have a recently consumed meal to use as energy, so it is *more likely* to pull from the fat stored in your body as it's the only energy source readily available.

The Human growth hormone has increased secretion during fasted states (both during sleep and after a period of fasting). Combine this increased growth hormone secretion with the body using fat as its fuel, the decrease in insulin production (and thus increase in insulin sensitivity), and you're essentially priming your body for muscle growth and fat loss with intermittent fasting.

Intermittent fasting can help teach your body to use the food it consumes more efficiently, and your body can learn to burn fat as fuel when you deprive it of new calories to constantly pull from (if you eat all day long). It does not necessarily mean that you will be hungry all day long. Fasting, in fact, some studies say, has a hunger depressing effect!

Drinking water, coffee or even tea during fasting is a wonderful way to prevent feeling very hungry. Try adding a dash of milk into your tea or coffee to make it better. You can make yourself a cup of herbal tea with one cinnamon stick, cloves, ginger and a pinch of tea leaves. Garnish them with fresh basil leaves and top it up with some natural honey! Best way to say thank you to your body.

While the fasting period can be very difficult at the beginning, the cherry on the cake is once the fasting is over, you can feast on during the eating window of your routine. Within this window, you can fit in 2 or 3 meals depending upon your love for food <3... However, the routine requires you to stick to certain rules try to avoid high-calorie intake and less sugary substances. Idea is to ensure that your body's insulin response system doesn't get activated. That'll just kill the benefits of fasting and the many hours you fasted to get to this point. What a shame!

You can have high protein food in the form of grills or stakes which will provide a balanced diet to your body to recover from the absence of nutrition for a while. Given that, I suggest you don't break your fast with a carb-heavy meal. Again, don't crank it up into overdrive suddenly. Ease it in.

When breaking a fast, the best thing to start with is a salad. Put some pasta in it if you're craving carbs. But don't go for a heavy sandwich or a burger or such. Brown rice can be a good start if you really need a heavy meal followed by some grilled or tossed veggies and black beans which is quite a nutrition-packed meal on its own. Soup can give you a good start too as it will hydrate your body too and keep it refreshing. Fruit lovers are my favorites as I'm one of them and I find ways to include fruits in my every meal. May it be a smoothie or a fruit salad or fruit custard. Adding fruits into your cereal can be a very colorful start to your day if you are eating breakfast within your intermittent fasting period. Oh, how can I skip seafood! As delicious as they taste, they are rich in minerals and protein with the right kind of fat that our body absolutely needs. May it be curry based or a grilled filet with lemon drizzled on top. Go ahead be creative.

Basically, have fun on your feast time to make this intermittent fasting journey a success. Y'know, Coz that's what the soul needs.

CONCLUSION

P.S. No matter what you do, don't forget to feel proud of your body. Always think the best for both your body and your soul and in turn, you will be thanked every moment of your life.

BEST OF LUCK!

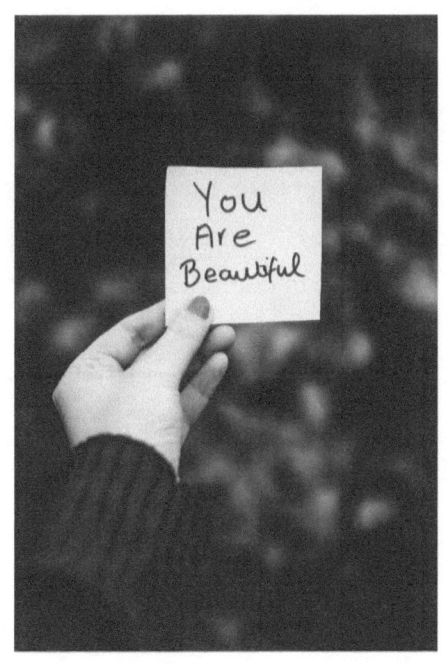

Can I Ask A Favour?

If you found this book, useful or otherwise then I'd really appreciate it if you would post a short review on Amazon. I do read all the reviews personally so that I can continually write on this subject.

Or please write to me at garciaofelda@gmail.com. I will respond in a day or two.

Thanks for your support.

Ofelda Garcia